I Fight for ...
Understanding

31 Days of Coping With
Huntington's Disease

GINNIEVIVE PATCH

ISBN: 10: 1545534632
ISBN-13: 978-154553463

For all the caregivers
    who help their loved ones through the journey
        of Huntington's disease and Juvenile Huntington's disease,
one day at a time,
    learning they possess strength and resilience
        they never knew they had
until they ended up on the HD/JHD roller coaster
    and had to hang on
        for the twisting, wild ride of their lives

ABOUT THE AUTHOR

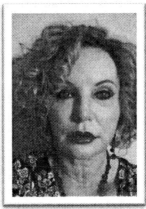

Ginnievive Patch (alias) grew up in southern California, born in Anaheim and raised in the mountains and High Desert until the age of 24, when she and her husband moved to Sacramento. Then, at age 28, they moved to Missouri. She and her ex-husband went to the same high school and re-met after high school and got married. She is the mother of three handsome, talented young men, two of whom have tested positive.

She started out in medicine at age twelve, volunteering as a candy striper, then worked her way up from working in a pharmacy, to getting her MA, to getting her RN. She has a background in family practice, lab, pediatric practice, psychology, oncology, and, for the last decade, medical aesthetics, including stem cells.

She ran a local Huntington's support group until her mother-in-law, Nana, who is in the end stages of HD, moved in with them. Currently, her home is open to caregiver spouses who need respite and peace to recharge.

She and her ex-husband, who has HD, have participated in HD research, along with their youngest son, who goes every year to Iowa University for the HD-Kids study. Her passion is to educate caregivers and help them survive the turmoil HD/JHD can cause in the early stages, primarily if the psychiatric symptoms outweigh the physical symptoms. She and her ex-husband remain close, making memories.

HD/JHD is a wild roller coaster, and her goal is to make the ride smoother for others.

Her motto is, "If I can help one family avoid being shredded apart, then I have accomplished my goal."

Ginnievive Patch

FOREWORD

If you are a caregiver for someone with Huntington's or Juvenile Huntington's disease, the image on the cover will immediately resonate with you.

How many times have we all heard a caregiver say, "Well, we're back on the roller coaster again!"

The roller coaster is a metaphor not just for the ups and downs of living with HD/JHD, but also for the breakneck speed and unpredictability with which changes often occur.

Just when we're riding along smoothly, things begin to build up, and just when they reach their peak, we plunge with our loved one into the abyss that always seems to be waiting just over the top.

But it doesn't end there. Everything levels out again, and we rock along, only to hit the rise, peak, and plunge once again. Over and over, we ride the roller coaster with our loved one who has HD/JHD, and every time, it can be just as scary and unpredictable as it was at the beginning of the ride because, you see, we never know what's coming around that blind corner!

A couple of years ago, Ginnievive Patch, who is a nurse, decided to write and post on a Facebook caregivers' group a coping tip for each day in May—Huntington's Disease Awareness Month. The tips herein are the ones she has so generously shared with us—31 in all—wisdom that comes from her experience of caring for her mother-in-law, her ex-husband, and two sons with HD.

We hope these tips will help you grab hold of the bars as you ride the roller coaster! Hang on, because you're in for one hell of a ride.

~ *Sharon McClellan Thomason*

Ginnievive Patch

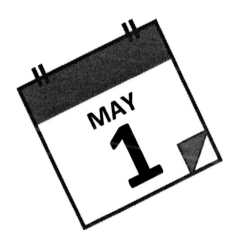

FIRST DAY OF HD/JHD AWARENESS MONTH!

Did you know that genetic variants on chromosomes 15 and 8 could hasten HD onset by 6 to 1.6 years respectively? Or that expression of a separate variant on chromosome 15 could delay onset by 1.4 years?? Also, the genetic study MTHFR can reveal genetic issues that can increase the severity of the psychiatric symptoms if the person is positive for the MTHFR mutation and is C677T and A1298C homozygous. People with the MTHFR mutation have a difficult time processing folate and folic acid. The result can be deficiencies in Folate, B6, and B12, all of which can affect a person's psychiatric health.

http://wellnessmama.com/27148/mthfr-mutation/

Ask to have the MTHFR test done on your loved one. It's a simple cheek swab that's sent off to a lab. If your loved one is positive, the MTHFR mutation can be treated with supplements. Your loved one's doctor may not even be aware of this test, so it's up to you to be your loved one's advocate.

Purple and blue are the colors of JHD and HD; wear them every day this month to advocate for your loved one!

Ginnievive Patch

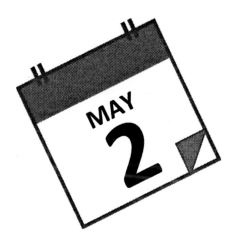

KIDS AS CAREGIVERS

This is a subject no one wants to talk about. It is also the one most easily overlooked. Children and teenagers are often involved in caregiving for a parent or grandparent or sibling with HD/JHD. It could be simple tasks such as wheeling Daddy to the table for dinner or helping to feed Sister. Ones who are not old enough to drive may be asked to sit with a loved one while the primary caregiver does errands or goes for a walk to recharge. Teenage girls sometimes are asked to help with bathing and dressing Mom, boys with Dad.

It is not wrong to ask a child to help, but it does cause them to grow up very quickly, and it can also mean that the illness leaves the child in the shadows because life is not about innocent childhood games and fairy tales; instead, it is about rearranging life around a sick loved one.

Sometimes, once kids are in their teens (and sometimes even younger), they can become overwhelmed once they realize their own risk.

Kids need to have support groups, too. A place that is not really about HD but about having fun and bonding with others in the same boat. HDYO (Huntington's Disease Youth Organization) offers free camps for kids ages 15-23 who live in the U.S., Canada, or Puerto Rico. Information can be found at https://en.hdyo.org/.

3

Venting is so important. My youngest son would sometimes come home from summer camp, and he would cry because his friends had "normal" dads. He admitted to feeling awkward when his friends saw Nana.

So let's remember to keep them recharged. Make sure their schools are educated about what they are living with. If we as caregivers get overwhelmed, imagine how a child feels.

Purple and blue. It is up to you! Truly, it is up to you.

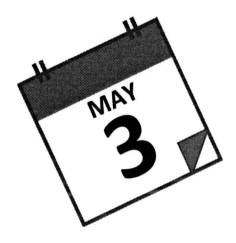

TEXTBOOK VS. REAL LIFE

Ever feel like you know more about HD/JHD than the neurologist? THAT is because you probably do. YOU are living it. You are there day to day, seeing the subtle and obvious changes. That is why reading every book, leaflet, and Internet site is so important to our quest. Read the boring medical books, read the fiction books, read the awareness flyers, and read the autobiographies.

A partial list includes *The Woman Who Walked Into the Sea* (Alice Wexler), *Mapping Fate* (Alice Wexler), *Someone Else's Life* (Katie Dale), *All Within: The Internal Journey of Huntington's Disease* (Susan E. Lawrence), *When Given Lemons* (Lauren Holder), *Ferris Wheel* (Katie Jackson), *Hurry Up and Wait* (Jimmy Pollard), *The Prayer of a Lifetime* (James V. D'Ambola, Jr., *Inside the O'Briens* (Lisa Genova), and *Life Interrupted* (published by Help 4 HD International).

Attend as many family conferences as you can. Put attending an annual HD Conference or Education Day on your bucket list to go to at least once (working on that myself). Sharing with others in the same boat has become the best teaching tool I can think of. Just ask the question, "Is this normal?" and I guarantee you will hear the word "YES!!!" over and over. Then you can sigh with relief that you are not alone, and you can take that information to your doctor.

Purple and blue, it is up to you.

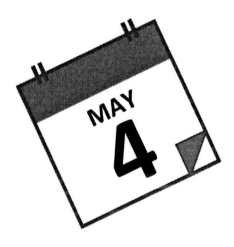

SAFETY FIRST

HD/JHD brings its own whirlwind of things that become dangerous, from eating to toileting to getting the flu, to violence, to falls, to pouring milk into a glass.

When a child is born, we run through our home, attaching safety locks, safety plug covers, removing sharp corner ends, blocking off stairways, yada, yada, yada. However, when a loved one with HD/JHD gradually gets clumsier, has trouble swallowing, cannot keep his/her balance, has outbursts, tries to continue in fields of work using dangerous tools, equipment, or vehicles, it is very hard to know what independence to eliminate.

We want our loved ones to feel independent and valuable, but let's face it: there are times when we as caregivers have to put our collective foot down. Intervention may be needed for driving, using glassware, starting a pureed diet.

ALL caregivers MUST take CPR and learn to do the Heimlich maneuver. YOU MUST.

We also have to set boundaries and protect our loved owns. Safe proof the house. Call 911 if you and/or your children are in danger or if your loved one with HD/JHD is suicidal.

It may cause conflict, may make you feel like a heel, but let's face it; purple and blue bruises are not what we mean by wearing our colors! Safety above all else.

Purple and blue, it's up to you!

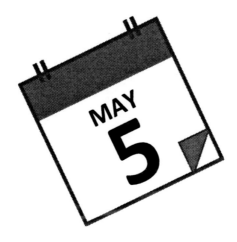

IMPULSIVITY AND NEGATIVITY

These are complicated symptoms of HD/JHD. They are also the ones that can get our loved ones and their families into the most trouble. The reason these two symptoms are so complicated is the fact that several things play into them.

The area of the brain that allows a person to gait emotion and to think logically and reasonably has eroded. The area that would allow you and me to hold our tongues when provoked, deny ourselves certain spending opportunities or sexual encounters, be polite to others in lines and in a store, patiently consider others in our choices is simply not there anymore.

Other things play into this as well. Our loved ones are dealing with grief, fear, shame, loss of self, loss of talents; this can make them feel like, "I deserve this; I am ill." It can also cause them to be resentful of healthy family members. It can cause reckless behavior. It can cause them to become aggressive and abusive. It can also cause them to become so depressed and angry at the world that at moments, they just do not care.

No two people handle the stress the same way, and people with HD have a physiological cause for not being able to handle stress. This

9

does not mean we sit back and let them do whatever they feel like doing, especially with kids involved, but it can give us better coping tools to understand the complexity of behavior. Perhaps most importantly, we can remind ourselves that it is the disease, not the person, talking or acting.

Compassion. Understanding. Respect. Unconditional love.

These are the lessons purple and blue teach us.

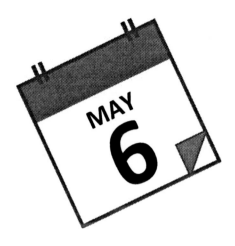

ST? OT? HD? JHD?

How do these letters work together? Speech therapy and occupational therapy can help your loved one with HD/JHD preserve a better quality of life. Teaching new skills to compensate for skills lost will help life travel along in a more normal fashion. Speech therapists can help with swallowing issues, verbal issues, and other coping skills such as ways to communicate once speech is compromised or lost. Occupational therapy can assist in motor issues, balance, and many aspects of daily living skills that the rest of us give no thought to.

Many simple things like thickening liquids, tucking the chin while swallowing, adaptive medical devices, etc. can be used to help our loved ones feel more independent. One thing I might add: if you are feeding a loved one with swallowing issues, and his/her head and torso move constantly, one of the things I find helpful when feeding Nana is keeping her in her high-backed wheelchair, belted in. I then brace one hand gently on her shoulder, have her tuck her chin, and bring the spoon to her. This helps stabilize her movements so she can focus just on swallowing.

Purple and blue, the things we must do.

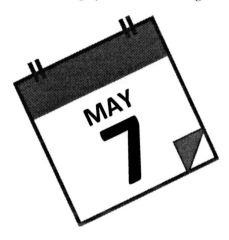

EVER HEARD THE TERM "FOLIE À DEUX"?

"Folie à deux" is a French term for shared psychosis. This is a rare mental illness where one person gets pulled into the delusions of another. Although rare, there is a risk of families with HD (and sometimes JHD) falling into this.

It may be subtle, simply starting to believe the things your loved one believes are reality, such as it is everyone else's fault at work, or maybe believing others are trying to sabotage your loved one, all the way to believing that the healthy person is crazy, the house is haunted, they are being watched, someone is trying to kill them, etc.

Spouses who are very close, where one is the caregiver and one is sick, are at the greatest risk for this rare occurrence. It is usually resolved with time apart. The more isolated a couple becomes due to illness, the greater the risk. The risk is particularly high when the one without HD struggles with depression, anxiety, bipolar disorder, etc., or comes from a family that "victimizes" its children, creating too much dependence, or in co-dependent relationships involving drugs and alcohol. It is a rare risk, but an ugly one.

Take care of yourself. Spend time away to recoup. Seek counseling. Read, read, read.

Purple and blue, caregivers; at times, it needs to be about you. Let us all stay emotionally healthy so that our loved ones have a fortress of love.

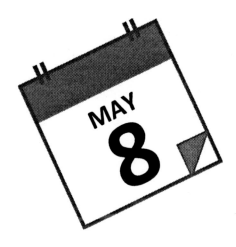

ABUSE

I have written on abuse before, but yes, I am gonna beat the dead horse again. SOOOO we all know HD/JHD causes the brain to literally deteriorate and die. We all know that people with HD/JHD lose control. But! What about hitting, screaming, threatening to kill us, and making life, well, a freaking nightmare? We can justify it by saying, "God, he/she has HD; this is all HD; I have to cope!" But do you???

A toddler can have a major tantrum, but is it okay? NO. We set boundaries for this immature behavior, and let's face it; your HD victim is now, figuratively, a toddler. YOU HAVE TO SET BOUNDARIES!!!! DID I STUTTER? UMMMMM, NOOO, I REPEAT: YOU HAAAAAAVVVVVVEEEEEE TO SET BOUNDARIES.

It is NOT okay for your loved one to abuse you. It is not okay for your loved one to abuse you. IT IS NOT OKAY FOR YOUR LOVED ONE TO ABUSE YOU. WAS THAT LOUD ENOUGH????????????? Good. You are awake.

15

HD is an illness that causes the brain to lose control. The centers for empathy, logic, and constraint are gone.

So it is okay to be hit, right? It is ok to be yelled at, right? Nope. Toddlers have brains not yet developed in these areas, so what do we do with them? We do not give them audience. We discipline them. We set boundaries.

This is what you do as well with your loved one who has HD. He or she is your toddler throwing a tantrum. You are the adult. Lay down the law. Call the law if necessary. It's hard to do, especially the first time, especially if you have to call the law, but sometimes it's the only way to keep you AND your loved one safe.

YOU ARE THE ADULT!!! Your HD victim is no longer qualified for the position. Is that cold? Cruel? NOPE!!! It is logical. Sane. It is what must be. Roles have reversed. YOU take the lead. YOU take control. Why???? You are the sane and logical one, and do not, do not, do not second guess yourself. Ever. HD makes people illogical, unreasonable, and unempathetic.

Trust your gut. You are right. They are out of control. Trust YOUR gut. Um, trust your gut. Did I mention? TRUST YOUR GUT!!!!

Purple and blue, it's all up to you!

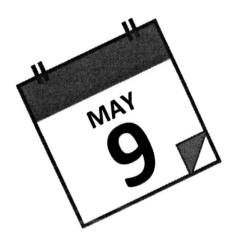

ADVOCACY

So many folks are becoming HD/JHD advocates, and nothing makes me more proud. It is getting easier to find genuine support and real life feedback not only from caregivers, but also from those living it! It does not matter what you do, whether it is buying books, t-shirts, and bracelets from each other or writing books, teaching classes, holding conferences and education days and symposia, and making videos. It is ALL important, and the word is getting out there!

We have folks getting buildings lit up in purple and blue; we have people making videos; we have grandkids designing t-shirts; we have stores and groups and education courses being taught all over the world.

Some books for folks who have only just learned about HD: *Life Interrupted* (published by Help 4 HD), *Me and HD* (Sarah Parker Foster), *It Is Better to Laugh Than Cry* (Clarence Vos), *The Hummingbird* (Deborah Goodman), *Learning to Live With Huntington's Disease: One Family's Story* (Sandy Sulaiman). There are so many more. Read as many as you can, share them, and know that you are not alone! Maybe everyone in your support group can read the same book and then discuss it.

Purple and blue, it is literally up to you!

Ginnievive Patch

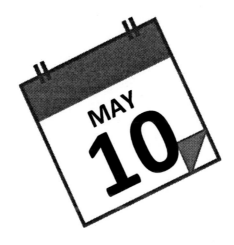

CAREGIVER SUPPORT FOR HD/JHD

Caregivers are truly a special breed of folks with incredible compassion, patience, and endurance. It is so hard when people in public stare or make rude comments about those we love.

Nana had been a stunning beauty in her youth and is now reduced to an unintelligible, shaking, toothless bag of bones, and as cruel as that sounds, I still see that beautiful, classy lady, and it breaks my heart when others look at her like a monster.

For those with children who have JHD, watching a young child who was once a bubbly, beautiful baby and cheerful, adventurous child with lots of friends slowly change and struggle even to walk and swallow, slowly become isolated into a world filled with doctors, nurses, feeding tubes, and wheelchairs instead of roller skates, bicycles, and prom clothes, nothing hurts a parent more. Nothing. Parents as caregivers sometimes are dealing with multiple sick family members in multiple stages.

Are you overwhelmed reading this? Think of living it. Most caregivers become the sole source of income, and the stress can take a huge toll on them, mentally and physically. Inner turmoil to not just run for the hills is real. So what is the solution? Support groups, both physical ones and online ones. Meeting up with other caregivers in person just to hug and say, "I understand," or "Yes, that is normal," can make a world of difference.

In addition to this, swapping ideas about medical devices and equipment, recipes for puréed diets, safety and financial tips allows us to face reality. We know a whole lot more about symptoms than the specialists do. We live it. Day in, day out. Even those caregivers who care from afar can tell the docs a thing or two.

Do not get me wrong; Centers of Excellence for HD are the best integrated teams there are for good care, but they mostly care for the victim, not the caregiver. So if you have not joined anything online or in person, do so. Take care of your own health—physical and mental. It's okay to take an antidepressant. It's okay to take time to do something just for yourself. I think for JHD parents this is crucial to giving your child the best outcome.

Schools can be educated, as can friends and family and babysitters, through support group efforts. Even police officers must be educated to avoid abuse.

You wear purple, I wear blue because supporting each other is up to me and you.

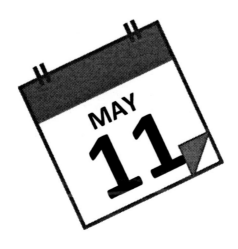

FOR THOSE IN HEAVEN

Over the past couple of years, we have lost so many to HD and JHD. Let us always remember them and their struggles. Some people release purple or blue balloons to mark their loved one's heavenly birthday or angelversary. Others set up foundations to help raise money for research or for family relief funds. Still others become much more active in advocacy.

Quality of life is so horrible at the end and in the final moments. As many of our children at risk or with JHD get older, time becomes more urgent. Time is a luxury we don't have. Today, I implore you to go to HD Trial Finder and enroll your loved one in a study. There are so many clinical trials going on today, more than at any time in history. Go to www.hdtrialfinder.org.

Purple and blue, the cure is up to you.

Ginnievive Patch

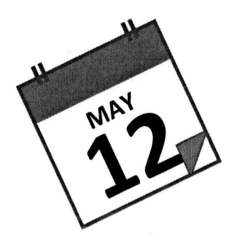

SEX

So today, I have pondered and fretted and reflected on what to say. The uncomfortable, ugly topic of promiscuity and sexual inappropriateness and obsession has come up in the support groups.... it is not pretty, but it is the one topic that can cause the most harm and can shred families to bits.

A man I once knew, who has HD, has gone to prison multiple times for sexual assault, child rape, and the list is long. Families are shredded over affairs outside the relationship because understanding this as a symptom and discussing it with a doctor is humiliating.

This does not happen to everyone with HD, but it does happen to a BIG portion of them. It hurts. It is risky behavior, putting spouses at risk for low self-esteem, STDs, and paranoia. We ALL want to trust the one we love to be faithful. But HD causes a loss of inhibitions. It also causes obsessive thinking, loss of impulse control, perseveration, and, for some, very hyperactive sexual desire and NO WAY to gait that.

As horrible as it really is on spouses, and yes, it is, it really is an HD symptom. A treatable one, IF your loved one is open to meds. The good news is it is usually a symptom that fades as the illness progresses, but alerting your doctor right away is crucial. This does not

23

mean you brush it aside. I can think of no more humiliating thing than having to get tested for STDs because of a cheating, out-of-control loved one. Sometimes, it can take the form of child molestation. Sometimes, it can be a new-found obsession with pornography or even child pornography.

Trust me; it really is the HD. Your loved one is succumbing to symptoms that may lead them to confusion, guilt, and very dangerous behavior.

On the flip side, some folks with HD lose ALL interest in sex. This, too, can be painful to partners. This, too, can stem from the depression, anxiety, and body changes brought on by HD. The person afflicted may really be suffering with low self-image. So HD has some really ugly, really painful symptoms.

Purple and blue. The unseen, untalked-about bruises.

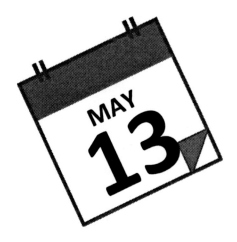

FINANCIAL AND EMOTIONAL PLANNING

Spend, spend, spend, yeah! Spend, spend, spend, yeah!

Out-of-control spending is a common occurrence in HD/JHD (if the child makes it into the teens or 20s). Bills and responsibilities seem to fly out the window while our loved ones accumulate mounds of senseless things. For one HD victim, it was shoes and guns; for my friend's loved one, it is eating takeout every day; for another, it is tools, eBay, Amazon, and vehicle upgrades, and, at one point, "toys" like trucks, trailers, boats, jet skis, and ATVs. For some, it is magazine subscriptions, clothes, lottery tickets, home decor, fabric, too many groceries, books, and the list can get very long.

This can be a source of fights and stress in an HD home, especially if you are already struggling financially. No matter how you reason with your loved one, write down the budget, agree on proper spending, do not be fooled. The area of the brain that thinks about consequences, that is reasonable, that allows one to have self-control has eroded.

This may mean that financial intervention may be necessary for a loved one who lives alone or even with someone. People with HD literally cannot handle money; they simply cannot quench that burning desire for immediate self-gratification. Add obsession, perseveration, inability to gait responses, and loss of executive function, then give them access to money, and yikes! It's a recipe for disaster. You may have to take away credit cards, debit cards, and check books. You may have to go to court and get conservatorship over your loved one. This will be a hard one because it is a slap in the face and signals loss of independence. Your loved one may get a little bitter at being treated "like a child," but well, let's face it, on many levels, he or she has "dematured." It is not the person's fault; it is just a fact of the disease.

If I could spare another family from the financial and emotional disaster that JHD/HD can cause, then I have done something worthwhile. My own family was financially impacted . However, what I learned from this is how important it is for me to help support other families, educating the young families on what to expect and how to avoid the mistakes we made. Planning for retirement, getting life insurance in place before testing, getting into group health insurance, and paying off your mortgage as early as you can will take a huge amount of stress off you in the future.

Join online and physical support groups. Also, seek counseling from others who have been there and done that, as well as professional counseling, ideally from an HD expert. Get an HD neurologist in place shortly after a positive test, and remember to also get regular checkups for yourself. It is your health that is on the line, too.

THEN, do not wait on the bucket list. Sit down with your loved one and plan for happy, memorable moments. There are organizations like Make-a-Wish Foundation that will help dreams on your loved one's bucket list come true. Time is short for HD/JHD families, and the future holds lots of change and chaos and painful moments. Savor the good ones. Write down the good moments. Take lots and lots of pictures. Maybe, just maybe, if these things are considered, I can help your family, and the future will be brighter.

Purple and blue. It is up to me to be here for you.

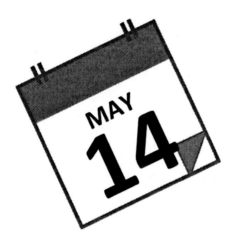

WHEN YOUR CHILD IS SICK

The worst words a parent ever hears are, "Your child has JHD," or, "Mom and Dad, I tested positive for HD."

I remember when my middle son's test results came in, we had no idea how to go through the proper channels. We knew next to nothing about this illness. His pediatrician called and gave us the news. It was good and bad. It was gene positive, as was his MRI for changes in the HD area of the brain, but it was not Juvenile HD.

Then when our youngest son turned 18, he was determined to get tested. Even though I felt he should wait to finish college, I was supportive of his choice and proud of his determination. He, too, tested positive.

What happened from there is that these two sons have become extra close. Their bond makes me smile. They "get" each other. I am very proud of them because they are open and honest about HD. They do not let it hold them back. They joke about it. They participate in research. I think if it were me, I could never be as brave.

So this month, wear purple and blue to honor our children who have the gene. They are our most cherished warriors.

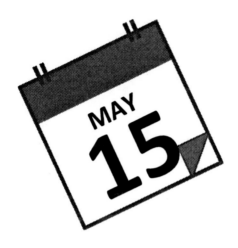

AN ABSENT LOVED ONE

What if your loved one seems vacant and unobservant, and just sits and does nothing? This can be a very complex symptom, too. One reason is that the ability to initiate is lost. Some of the brain changes cause apathy. To compound that, depression can cause a debilitating lack of interest. Third, reasoning, problem solving, forward thinking, and judgement are lost.

The face may become mask-like (called a flat affect), lacking expression other than twitching and grimacing. This may lead others in the family to feel that the person with HD no longer cares for them, or is being lazy or selfish.

I find with Nana, keeping a calendar in her room helps. Routine helps, as does asking questions that are not open ended. Initiate conversation with your loved one, but do not expect long answers. Don't expect them to initiate conversation. Tell your loved one ahead of time when the routine is going to change. It is lonely, sitting and not talking or being talked to. That deadpan expression, sitting like a zombie, and paying no attention to anything other than what is right in front of them are ALL HD/JHD.

Take time to pull them out of it. If I say to Nana, "Look at those beautiful flowers," she will lift her head, focus on them, and see them for the first time, even though they are right in front of her. Then she enjoys them.

Purple and blue. Sad, but true.

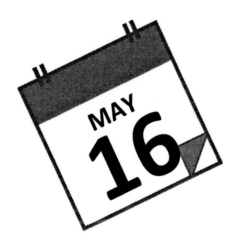

SHARK EYES

"I can see it in their eyes." Way back, before I knew much about HD at all, I noticed this look in certain family members' eyes. I noticed them turn their whole heads to look at something off to the side. Then after meeting other people outside the family who also had HD, I noticed the same exact look.

What is it???? Well, there is a dent in the visual saccades. With neuronal loss, tracking and spatial perception are off. It may actually be a very subtle early symptom.

We had a police officer stop us once at a routine checkpoint over a holiday, and he asked my husband if he had ever had a head injury. This was years before diagnosis, but the officer noticed that his tracking was off. It is not your imagination when you think you see a change in their eyes. It is a true symptom. You can read more about it here: http://www.ncbi.nlm.nih.gov/pubmed/9425536

Purple and blue, the symptom is true.

Ginnievive Patch

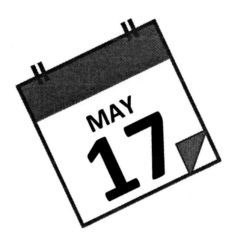

SUPER STRENGTH

Does it seem like your loved one has the might of Hercules? Even the tiniest HD/JHD victim can break couches, pull towel bars off the wall, break toilet seats and dining room chairs, pull cabinet doors right off the wall, and pull his/her caregiver over while being helped up.

This comes about for several reasons. A healthy central nervous system signals to our muscles to gradually support our weight as we sit down; it signals us to gently open a cabinet, shut a drawer, or pull a towel off the bar. For someone with HD/JHD, not only do involuntary movements interfere, but the neuron signals that help us control purposeful movements are delayed or even destroyed. This actually comes in handy when getting a bear hug because Nana can squeeze the daylights out of me.

The best way to handle this is two-fold: one, occupational therapy can help, along with physical therapy and exercise; also, doing small things like getting assistive medical devices like chairs that lift, raised toilet seats, bars for the tub and showers, etc. can help. Do not get angry at your superheroes. Like Superman, they cannot control their strength.

Look, what was that purple and blue flash that just obliterated the couch? It is our purple and blue superheroes; it is true!

33

Ginnievive Patch

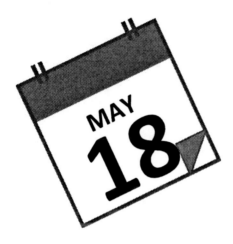

ANOSOGNOSIA

What does that mean? Anosognosia is an organic disorder that comes with HD/JHD. It is a multifaceted disorder caused by changes in the brain. It may seem like denial, but it's not. It is literally unawareness. It may first be noticed by loved ones as an inability for the person with HD to see or notice his/her own involuntary movements, cognitive decline, or psychiatric symptoms. I do not know how many times my loved one has asked, "What symptoms do I even have?"

In the book *Learning to Live with Huntington's Disease*, the author was shocked when a coworker said she should not wear bracelets because it was distracting students, due to her movements. She also did not recognize her difficult behavior; it was everyone else.

This also can leak into other sensory issues of smell, sight, hearing, taste, inability to identify an object or person. They may not recognize spills and therefore not clean them up. As the disease progresses, this lack of awareness can become more evident. The person may seem totally unaware of the environment, like walking into snow in shorts, not noticing the room around them unless pointed out, and trying to continue skills that have been lost.

You can read more about this puzzling symptom here: http://www.hddrugworks.org/dr-goodmans-blog/severe-anosognosia-like-walking-through

Purple and blue, they still know you!

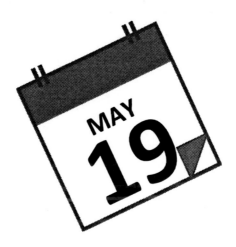

"GIVE ME THOSE KEYS, PLEASE"

This is one sentence that can cause total devastation to a person with HD or JHD. It is a milestone in the loss of independence, and it changes the dynamics of family logistics. This may mean that the responsibility to cart kids to and from school and practices and programs falls on the healthy spouse/parent. It means the sick person can no longer hop in the car to shop, go to work, run an errand. It kind of makes HD/JHD slap everyone in the face with, "I am here to stay."

It is a slippery slope and can cause World War Three at home because, due to anosognosia (see the May 18th entry), the person with HD may not even notice how he/she drives. HD can disrupt driving skills on so many levels, from the slow response time, poor judgement, poor impulse control to visual saccades and spatial perception, poor hand-eye coordination, inability to keep a consistent speed, slow reaction time, and involuntary movements of hands and feet. The list is a long, scary one. Please remember that these changes put other drivers on the road at risk as well as our loved one.

Some centers offer road test assessments for people with Huntington's disease.

A good source for more information about this is: http://web.stanford.edu/group/hopes/cgi-bin/hopes_test/driving-and-huntingtons-disease/

Purple and blue, I wish it weren't true.

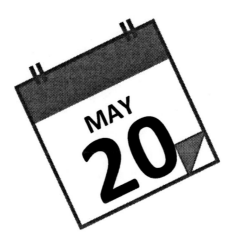

FEAR

One of the worst things about HD/JHD is the ripple effect and tidal wave the diagnosis causes. Once children learn they are at risk, fear can set in while watching a parent decline before their eyes. Fear.

A spouse can become terrified about losing the relationship, about the financial impact, about where to find proper help. Fear.

Parents can become hyper-vigilant regarding their children, watching every little thing with the constant, nagging fear in the back of their minds: is my child showing signs? Fear.

Just receiving news that your life is going to be cut short, but not before this monster slowly maims you. Fear alone in HD/JHD families can cause insurmountable hills of stress. That "OMG, what are we going to do now?" fear can thwart open, honest conversations about the illness in families.

Fear can cause those with HD or at risk to become secretive and withdrawn and to lash out at others. Fear can cause family members to not disclose a diagnosis. Fear can cause suicide. Fear can cause divorce. Fear can cause risky behavior. Fear can cause heavy, unmanageable grief.

One time we went to see my loved one's aunt. We knew she had HD but had not seen her in a while. To say that we were shocked at what we saw is putting it mildly. Once we left, my husband turned to me, pale, and said, "THAT scares the sh-- out of me." I squeezed his hand. All I could think of myself, as icy chills ran down my back, was fear. Afraid for my family.

Let us conquer fear by empowering each other with knowledge, support, and participation in research. Let's empower our communities by educating law enforcement, doctors, nurses, and nursing homes. Let's empower our children and teach them about family planning options, financial planning, and all aspects of the illness. Let us conquer fear.

Purple and blue. It is up to you.

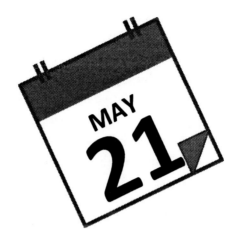

PURÉED FOOD
DOES NOT HAVE TO BE GROSS

Coming up with a creative diet for a loved one who has to be fed puréed foods can be a challenge. Getting proper nutrition in your loved one can really be tough when they need sooooo many calories to keep up with the metabolic changes of HD. (People with HD need 5,000 calories per day just to maintain their weight!)

There may be a point at which your family will opt for an abdominal port to supply liquid nutrition through a feeding tube (or, in a child, a g-button). In the meantime, puréeing foods and making them look nice can be tough. When swallowing issues first start, chopping foods finely and supplying slightly thicker liquids may be all that is needed.

A speech therapist can help you evaluate and meet your loved one's needs. Also, safety straws, although expensive, may help. These have a valve that only allows a certain amount of liquid in at a time. When my mother-in-law lived with me, I would literally just purée whatever we had and pour gravy and sauces on, being careful to use different colored foods and textures to make it look nice. We had ice cream and cheesecake for dessert often because she could eat that easily. Making broccoli, potatoes, etc. into thick cream soups helps, too. If pancakes are soaked in syrup, they seems to go down well. Scrambled eggs are a "normal" food they can usually eat. I used to add **protein powder to fruit smoothies, pancake mix, and soups for extra** calories and nutrition. Season the puréed foods exactly how you would your own food. Bland puréed food is gross, and remember that just as vision is affected, smell and taste can be, too.

At meal time, remember to keep the room fairly quiet, TV off, no music, and remind your loved one to tuck the chin. Distraction is not good for those who choke easily. Be creative with presentation. Giving a loved one mashed potatoes and oatmeal every day gets boring. This is a human being, and mealtime may be the only thing left to enjoy.

Purple and blue. Their nutrition is up to you.

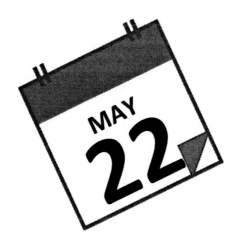

THE UGLY CHOICES

Nursing homes. When is that the option that must be chosen? Years ago, I would have looked down on folks who chose a nursing home. Yes, you read it right; that was YEARS ago, before I actually had my mother-in-law, who is end stage HD, live with us. HD/JHD are very taxing and time-consuming illnesses for the entire family.

If the kids are grown, and you are retired, it may be easier to keep a loved one home than when there are young ones running about who need to be carted to and from school and school functions. Kids are never quiet and keep a household in motion. Throw in a fulltime career and a very sick spouse and maybe also a JHD child, and life can become too much for one person as a caregiver to handle.

I was blessed as I was able to hire my own mom to stay with Nana during the day while I worked, and she helped with housework, but even then, if I was up all night cleaning up vomit and diarrhea with Nana, work the next day was difficult.

Folks with HD/JHD thrive on routine and a stable environment. They want what they want right now, and don't you dare rush them or make them wait! That, in and of itself, is tough. For my own family, the transition to a nursing home was made when other members of the household suffered. It seemed to cause a battle of wills among my early-stage man and his late-stage mom and our teenaged son as to who should receive priority. My own arthritis was making it murder to bathe and dress Nana and lift her chair in and out of a car. The constant **aggressive outbursts from my husband during this time and the suicidal** thoughts of my son made me finally choose to put Nana in a home. It was not easy, not what I wanted, but I had to think of my child.

Since then, my son has tested positive, along with my other son, and I can say the nursing home placement was the best solution for all of us. I see Nana often, still do her laundry and nails and feed her when I show up at mealtime. She looks forward to our visits. Her son enjoys her more.

A nursing home is not for everyone, and if your situation allows you to keep them home, then do so; however, when it becomes an emotional or physical danger to keep them home, look into a nursing home. Sometimes you can be a caregiver from a distance.

Purple and blue. When is a nursing home right for you?

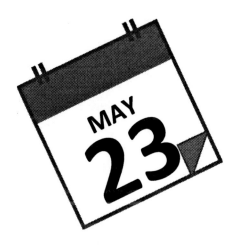

SPLISH, SPLASH,
I WAS TAKING A BATH ...

Oh, no, I was giving a bath to someone else with chorea! Bathing a loved one can be a huge challenge, especially if that person is larger than you. The whole scene usually consists of all arms and legs and water everywhere. Both the caregiver and patient with HD/JHD end up soaked.

One thing that helped us tremendously was a bath chair and a hand-held shower head in the tub. They make benches that sit over the edge and slide in so you can seat the person with HD/JHD and then scoot him/her into the tub. If you cannot find one of those, having a handrail attached on the side of tub and also on the wall of the tub helps, too. Another solution is a Hoyer lift, purchased from medical supply companies.

Even though bathing is a very intimate and loving gesture, it can also become a battle of wills. I actually had to make a bath schedule for Nana because she would often say, "I do not need a bath," so we just made certain days of the week bath days. I really would have preferred every day because when an adult is in diapers, skin integrity

45

and odor are a problem, so I also kept a box of antibacterial baby wipes in the restroom to keep the genital area clean. I often had to sneak out the dirty clothes and start the machine lickity split so she would not drag the dirty clothes back out.

Hygiene (or lack of!) usually becomes an issue at some point in HD/JHD, and your loved one may not notice if body odor gets offensive. It can be especially challenging if your loved one doesn't yet need help with bathing. For those who have lost that ability, bath time can be a time of bonding for both of you. Take your time with them, wash their hair, laugh, dry them carefully, apply deodorant and body lotion, and dry and style their hair. Nana and I took this time to also do her nails and to just help her feel fresh and human.

This is also a good time to inspect for bruises and injuries they may not tell you about and to make sure the skin is not breaking down anywhere.

Purple and blue, you get a shower, too!

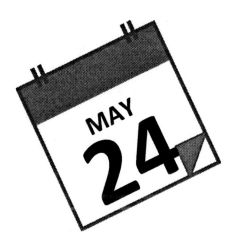

PHONE CALLS

My cell phone rings several times a day. It is the nursing home, Nana wanting to know when I am coming. She cannot handle running out of pie or Reese's. She panics that I won't come. I work full time and cannot answer every call.

Several factors play into these repeated phone calls: perseveration, loneliness, forgetfulness (forgot she just called an hour ago), fear, obsession, impulsiveness, and lack of awareness of others. She sees her Reese's are getting low. She has lost all conception of time and does not realize her calendar is marked and has a week to go. She wants me to remember Reese's. I never forget them. She wants me to visit. I always do. The only thought in her mind is, "My Reese's are low; I have to tell Ginnie; she has to bring Reese's; I am low on Reese's; I have to tell Ginnie."

That thought will not leave her mind. HD/JHD causes this symptom (perseveration). Nana cannot help it. Think of it in terms of a newborn baby. The baby is hungry. The baby wants to be fed. The baby wants to be fed now. So the baby cries until someone feeds the baby. An infant loves you. An infant recognizes you, but an infant cannot look at you and think, "Oh, Mom is working; she comes at home at 6; I will get fed at 6:15."

Nope, not gonna happen. Our loved ones begin to think in this same way as the illness progresses. It is neuronal loss. It cannot be helped. This is sometimes a difficult thing for caregivers, but you would never be mad at an infant or think him/her selfish.

Purple and blue, we care for you.

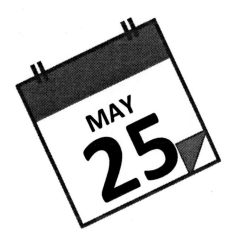

WHAT ABOUT THE CHILDREN?

HD/JHD can cause problems for school children. Remember that their situation is so different from their friends. Sick parents may not be able to attend all school functions, and the child may feel embarrassed by the sick parent who looks "different" and awkward around kids with "normal" parents. A parent may show up to pick up a child, or for a school function, and the school personnel may think the parent is drunk. They may even call the police. People (yes, even adults!) may make fun of the unusual movements of the sick parent.

To help ease all of this, it is good to ask for an assembly and to educate the kids and adults of the school about HD/JHD in an age-appropriate way. Encouraging and allowing kids to join an HD youth organization is helpful, too. Two such organizations are HDYO (Huntington's Disease Youth Organization) and NYA (National Youth Alliance).

Kids with JHD may end up becoming excluded from things, like parties, as the illness progress. Once kids know, though, that a child needs their help and has an illness, or is worried about a parent who has an illness, you would be surprised at how quickly kids adapt and try to include him/her. Children have an amazing capacity for compassion, and it is no longer scary if they understand what is wrong.

49

Education is key, and in some school systems, there is even extra support for kids who are dealing with chronic trauma. Ask about resources that are offered by the school.

If your child is at risk or has JHD, he or she will need an IEP (Individual Education Plan) that outlines all the accommodations and modifications that need to be made for your child to succeed in school. This may come in the form of counseling, shortened school days, individual aides, a quiet place and extended time for testing. The possibilities are endless.

Don't be afraid to speak up for your child. You know your child better than anyone else, and you are his/her fiercest advocate! Ask other parents what they have done in similar situations, and if appropriate, add those things to your bag of tricks.

Purple and blue, the painful things we need to do.

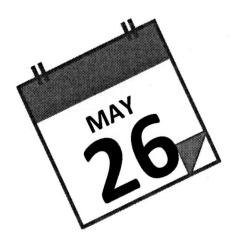

CAREGIVERS

I am packing up to move to a different house! For two days, though, I have done nothing, I mean nothing, but think about caregivers for HD/JHD. These are the folks who go unnoticed and who give up their entire lifestyle to take care of loved ones. These folks often become both mother and father. Nurse and advocate. Maid and taxi driver. Counselor and pupil. They often go unheard. Their own health and mental health often come second, third, maybe not at all. Suicide among caregivers can be as high as those with the illness. So let's talk about these folks.

Who are they???? Often it is a spouse, sibling, child, parent, partner of someone ill. Who is caring for them? They often have to work full time and care for a family, on top of caring for a sick one. These folks work 24/7, and many have NO relief. I was lucky. I could hire my mom to stay with Nana while I worked, because Nana had a pension. Not everyone has that. Even then, no one was there to stay up at night with me when she would vomit and have diarrhea. I was met at the door every night after 8- to 14-hour work days with the question, "What is for dinner?" before I could even get the door closed behind me.

Caregivers often go without sleep, often because the loved one who's sick is up all night, with days and nights "turned around." Caregivers often suffer verbal abuse. Caregivers often suffer isolation. Caregivers are the ones who worry about the kids at risk, the hospital bills, the competency of health care workers. They go unnoticed. Who calls the caregiver and says, "Hey, do you need a break? How are you holding up?"

This is because HD and JHD are LOOOOOOONG, drawn-out illnesses that often make the outside world get bored with caring. When there are no physical symptoms, there may be no offers to help because the disease is "invisible." It may be all dedication at first, but then the years toil on.

When you need it, learn to ask for help from friends and family if they ask, "What can I do?" Put aside your pride. Ask for help with cooking, cleaning, shopping, transportation, the things we're so afraid to "bother" other people with.

So today, my prayer is for the ones holding down the fort.

Purple and blue. I salute you.

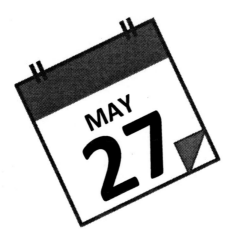

GUILT AND GRIEF

Sometimes the words, "I hate you," slip across our brains. We hate what the person we love has become. We hate what HD has done to our loved ones and what caregiving has done to us. Some of us may have "survivor's guilt" because we tested negative while other family members tested positive. We have moments of weakness. Anger. Exhaustion. We have moments when we really mess up and even mimic the hated actions of our loved ones.

Sometimes we reach out to others, anyone who will fill the void and have a normal conversation with us. Then we have moments of private grieving. Isolating ourselves. Pulling the sheets up over our heads. Sobbing for what the future brings. Broken. Fearful for our children. Feeling sooooo alone, so destroyed, sooo much like Atlas bearing the weight of the world.

I am here to tell you: you are not a bad person. Caregivers often experience types of grief known as anticipatory and ambiguous grief. You are not evil. YOU are human. Doing a really tough job. Taking on so much extra and wearing so many hats. We gather here for solace. We gather here to refresh, to vent, and to finally breathe, knowing others are in the same damn boat. This is where physical support groups and online support groups can make a huge difference.

Today, you are normal. Today, you are understood. Today, I am praying for you.

Purple and blue, today I love you and care about you.

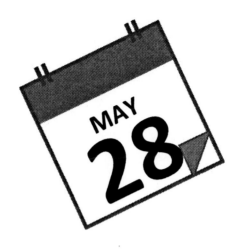

MASS DESTRUCTION

HD families with multiple family members sick with JHD and HD, others at risk and untested, all living under one roof, can be very stressful. Caregivers may find they have no time for themselves, and their own health may suffer. There can be multiple flames being thrown, like tantrums, doctor's appointments, school, work, changing diapers and feeding tubes, dressing self and many members of the family, feeding everyone, and then what if the caregiver needs to have a gallbladder out, or gets strep throat, or needs a knee replaced? Who cares for them and everyone else?

If you live in an area where hired help is available, then please make the call. If not, try networking with other families in your area to solicit help. Church members and extended family members who are not sick can help. Look into respite care. Even Hospice can offer assistance—and don't be afraid of Hospice. Some people remain on Hospice for YEARS. Do not try to do it all alone, even if it's hard for you to ask for help. This is an illness that truly takes a village because mental and physical isolation is real, and caregivers are humans who can get sick, too. If you don't take care of yourself, you won't be able to take care of anyone else.

Purple and blue; take care of YOU.

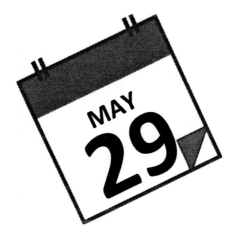

PURPLE AND BLUE HEARTS

It is ironic that May is HD/JHD Awareness Month. It is also Memorial Day month; Memorial Day is the last Monday of May. Two years ago, my father passed away on Memorial Day, which was also my birthday. He was a World War II Marine.

Unlike my ex-spouse's family, I had never heard of HD/JHD. I heard lots and lots about wars and soldiers and platoons and bombings. I heard all about the horrific things my father witnessed when their ship was attacked.

Now, I sit and ponder about folks with HD/JHD who may have served our country, only to have to come home after that service to fight a completely different war against an enemy we have no weapons for. My dad lived to be 93; HD/JHD folks sometimes don't see 18 or 50.

As I reach my 52nd birthday and reflect on my father's death, I realize how many in our community we have lost and how many will never live to be my age. They have lost the battle to HD/JHD, the bravest, bravest, strongest soldiers ever.

We have all heard of Purple Hearts. How about purple and blue hearts? To those of you who served our nation and gave us our freedom, I will fight to try and help you gain freedom from this enemy.

Purple and blue, I salute you.

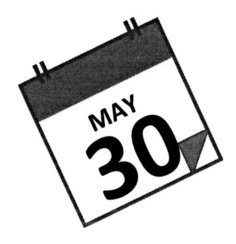

KIDS-HD AND KIDS-JHD

Today, I really want to talk about Kids-HD and Kids-JHD, programs that Dr. Peggy Nopoulos is conducting at the University of Iowa. This study uses children who are gene positive, children who are gene negative, and children with JHD. My youngest son has been in this research study for years, and the importance is truly significant in finding gene therapies for a cure.

Dr. Nopoulos and her team have learned that there are differences, even in childhood, between children with and without the mutated gene, EVEN if it is not JHD. I will tell you that my middle son had an MRI as an adolescent that already had changes in the HD area. He does have the gene, but not JHD. This intrigued Dr. Bradley Schlaggar at St. Louis Children's Hospital in Missouri, and he asked to keep a copy of the MRI.

If doctors and researchers can detect and understand how a young developing brain is affected, then early intervention could be key when finding a cure. Please, please look into enrolling your kids who are at risk or who have JHD in this study. All travel and lodging expenses are paid, and the child receives a stipend.

More information about this study can be found here:

https://medicine.uiowa.edu/psychiatry/research/kids-hd-and-kidsjhd.

To our littlest warriors, purple and blue, we salute you!

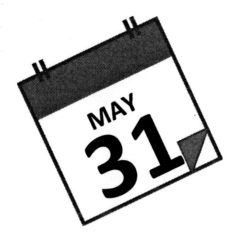

BLAMING GOD AND FINDING PEACE

Blaming God. Yep, I said that, and no, I am not pushing my religious beliefs on anyone. The fact is that some families are very religious and practice their faith together, and then one day your loved one stops wanting to participate in family faith and church activities, which can really cause division and stress.

On the flip side, it may be you as the caregiver who gets a little irked at God. I am just gonna be blunt. I have walked alone down dirt roads, screaming at God about how unfair He is. I have cried and pleaded with Him for negative results as my children got tested. I have held my ex while he cried and said, "What kind of God does this?" I have listened to him spit venomously, "God, don't give me this Christianity bullshit. If God is so good, this would not be happening."

You are not evil. Your loved one is not evil. You are not sinning. This is a normal human response. Some families become more faithful and closer to God, but many do not. Do not beat yourself up. Do not let other family members make you feel guilty. Blaming and questioning God is normal in the grieving process of HD/JHD. It really is.

One of the things that stands out, if you read very many books on HD/JHD, is the chaos and uproar the disease can cause. Rigid thinking, perseveration, anosognosia, depression, irrational thinking, inability to gait emotion, chorea, dysphagia, dysphasia, loss of inhibitions, obsession, lack of initiation, disorganized thinking, inability to handle stress, anger, explosiveness, delusions, hallucinations, inability to leave routine—and this list can get very, very long—can really shred families to bits.

It's hard to find peace. This is especially true in families that were either blindsided or who kept the family illness a secret. It is a well-documented fact that children who are well informed and educated on ALL aspects of the illness handle it better. Responsible adults who keep appointments with their neurologists, psychiatrists, and counselors do better than the ones who run and hide.

Finding peace in this raging war is difficult. Lower your expectations of your loved one who has HD/JHD. Do not expect him/her to respond the way he/she "should," or the way he/she used to, or the way you need him/her to respond because that person is gone. Bask in the lucid moments.

When my ex-husband and I are walking and talking and sharing a glass of wine, I cherish that, because maybe tomorrow he will hate me and find fault in me. He may call me horrible names and storm off and not contact me for weeks, months, or longer.

Know that the more you learn, the more your heart will be able to listen to your head. One of my caregiver friends says to herself during a crazy moment, "His proteins are folded, his proteins are folded." This keeps her emotions in check to handle her hubby. I like that.

Purple and blue, may peace find you.

All net proceeds from the sale of this book will go to
Help 4 HD International's Family Relief Fund,
which provides emergency assistance to families in crisis.

If you would like to make a donation to any of
Help 4 HD International's programs, please go to
www.help4hd.org.
Donations may be made via PayPal or credit/debit card.

Checks may be mailed to:
Help 4 HD International
5050 Laguna Blvd. 112 543
Elk Grove, CA 95758

If you would like to donate to a specific program,
please make a notation on your check.